How to Make

Natural Body Scrubs

Dr Miriam Kinai

ISBN: 1478101148

ISBN-13: 978-1478101147

Contents

1

Body Scrubs Making Equipment

Glass bowl

Wooden spoon

Glass jar

* * * * *

2

Basic Body Scrub Recipe Ingredients

A body scrub basically consists of the following 4 ingredients:

1. Exfoliant - this is the abrasive that gently removes the dead skin cells to reveal the smooth, glowing skin beneath. These can be divided into physical exfoliants and chemical exfoliants. Physical exfoliants include brown sugar, white sugar, sea salt, Epsom salt, baking soda, cornmeal, finely ground oatmeal, rice powder, apricot kernels, coffee beans and jojoba seeds. Chemical exfoliants include butter milk, yogurt, pineapple and papaya.

2. Vegetable oil - because most body scrubs use physical exfoliants, vegetable oils are added to make a soft paste for ease of application. In addition, they too have their own benefits such as skin nourishing vitamins. Perfect examples include sweet almond oil and olive oil.

3. Fragrance - these add a sweet aroma to the body scrub. Essential oils are used in natural body scrubs due to their healing aromas and therapeutic benefits. Grated lemon rind, cocoa and coffee are also used to scent body scrubs.

4. Colorant - these add visual appeal to the body scrub. Perfect examples of natural substances used to color body scrubs include turmeric, cinnamon, cocoa and coffee.

***

The following is a basic body scrub recipe

2 cups exfoliant such as brown sugar

¾ cup or 6 oz or 190 ml of vegetable oil such as olive oil

10-20 drops essential oil such as lavender essential oil

½ teaspoon colorant such as cocoa powder

* * * * *

3

Basic Body Scrub Instructions

1. Mix the exfoliant (in this case brown sugar) and the vegetable oil (in this case olive oil) in a glass bowl with a wooden spoon until they form a thick paste.

2. Add your fragrance (in this case lavender essential oils) drop by drop as you stir until you attain your required scent.

3. Add your colorant (in this case cocoa powder) pinch by pinch as you stir until you get an appealing color.

4. Pour your homemade handmade scrub into a glass jar and use as required.

* * * * *

4

Therapeutic Body Scrubs Recipes

Normal and Sensitive Skin Body Scrub Recipe

2 cups brown sugar

¾ cup or 6 oz or 190 ml of vegetable oils such as apricot kernel oil, sweet almond, and avocado oil.

10-20 drops essential oil such as Lavender essential oil

½ teaspoon colorant such as cocoa powder

Follow the above Basic Body Scrub Recipe Instructions.

***

Dry Skin Body Scrub Recipe

2 cups brown sugar

¾ cup or 6 oz or 190 ml of moisturizing vegetable oils used to manage dry skin such as sweet almond oil, sunflower oil, jojoba, avocado oil, apricot kernel, olive, evening primrose, virgin coconut, fractionated coconut oil, and calendula oil.

10-20 drops of essential oils used to manage dry skin such as Lavender, Roman chamomile, and Ylang ylang essential oils.

½ teaspoon colorant such as cocoa powder

Follow the above Basic Body Scrub Recipe Instructions.

***

Mature Skin Body Scrub Recipe

2 cups brown sugar

¾ cup or 6 oz or 190 ml of moisturizing vegetable oils such as sweet almond oil, sunflower oil, jojoba, avocado oil, apricot kernel, olive oil, evening primrose, virgin coconut, and calendula oil.

10-20 drops of Geranium essential oil.

½ teaspoon colorant such as cocoa powder

Follow the above Basic Body Scrub Recipe Instructions.

***

Cellulite Body Scrub Recipe

2 cups brown sugar

¾ cup or 6 oz or 190 ml of moisturizing vegetable oils such as sweet almond and olive oil.

10-20 drops of essential oils used to manage cellulite such as grapefruit, sweet orange, and geranium.

½ teaspoon colorant such as cocoa powder

1 teaspoon coffee grounds

Follow the above Basic Body Scrub Recipe Instructions.

***

Eczema Body Scrub Recipe

2 cups brown sugar

¾ cup or 6 oz or 190 ml of vegetable oils beneficial for the management of eczema such as Evening primrose oil, Rose hip oil, Cranberry seed oil, Calendula, Coconut oil, Sweet almond oil, Borage seed oil and Jojoba.

10-20 drops of essential oils used for eczema treatment such as Geranium, Lavender, Roman chamomile, and Rosemary essential oils.

½ teaspoon colorant such as cocoa powder

1 teaspoon dried ground herbs (optional) used to manage eczema such as calendula, chamomile, and St John's wort.

Follow the above Basic Body Scrub Recipe Instructions.

PS Don't use this scrub on red inflamed areas or active eczema lesions.

***

Psoriasis Body Scrub Recipe

2 cups brown sugar

¾ cup or 6 oz or 190 ml of vegetable oils beneficial for the management of psoriasis such as Evening primrose, Apricot kernel oil and Jojoba. Use olive oil if you do not have them.

10-20 drops of essential oils used for the management of psoriasis such as Roman chamomile, Tea tree, and Lavender essential oils.

½ teaspoon colorant such as cocoa powder

1 teaspoon dried ground herbs (optional) used to manage psoriasis such as chamomile flowers, and lavender flowers.

Follow the above Basic Body Scrub Recipe Instructions.

PS Don't use scrub on red inflamed areas or active psoriasis lesions.

***

Menopausal Symptoms Body Scrub Recipe

2 cups brown sugar

¾ cup or 6 oz or 190 ml of vegetable oils such as olive oil.

10 - 20 drops of essential oils used to manage menopausal symptoms such as Clary sage, Geranium, Lavender, Peppermint, Roman chamomile, and Rosemary essential oils.

½ teaspoon colorant such as cocoa powder

1 teaspoon dried ground herbs (optional) used for menopausal symptoms such as chamomile flowers and rosemary leaves.

Follow the above Basic Body Scrub Recipe Instructions.

***

Pre-Menstrual Tension (PMS) and Painful Periods Body Scrub Recipe

2 cups brown sugar

¾ cup or 6 oz or 190 ml of vegetable oils such as olive oil.

10 - 20 drops of essential oils used to manage menstrual symptoms such as Clary sage, Geranium, Lavender, and Roman chamomile essential oils.

1 teaspoon dried ground herbs (optional) such as lavender flowers and chamomile flowers.

½ teaspoon colorant such as cocoa powder

Follow the above Basic Body Scrub Recipe Instructions.

***

Stress Management Body Scrub Recipe

2 cups brown sugar

¾ cup or 6 oz or 190 ml of vegetable oils such as olive oil.

10 - 20 drops of essential oils used for managing stress such as Lavender, Roman Chamomile, Bergamot, Clary sage, Petitgrain, Geranium, Marjoram, Peppermint, Rose, Sandalwood, Ylang ylang essential oils.

1 teaspoon dried ground herbs (optional) used for managing stress such as lavender flowers and chamomile flowers.

½ teaspoon colorant such as cocoa powder

Follow the above Basic Body Scrub Recipe Instructions.

***

Sadness Body Scrub Recipe

2 cups brown sugar

¾ cup or 6 oz or 190 ml of vegetable oils such as olive oil.

10 - 20 drops of essential oils used for the treatment of depression such as Bergamot, Clary sage, Roman chamomile, Lavender, Rosemary, Rose, Ylang ylang.

1 teaspoon dried ground herbs (optional) used to manage depression such as rosemary leaves and St John's wort.

½ teaspoon colorant such as cocoa powder

Follow the above Basic Body Scrub Recipe Instructions.

***

Mental Exhaustion Body Scrub Recipe

2 cups brown sugar

¾ cup or 6 oz or 190 ml of vegetable oils such as olive oil.

10 - 20 drops of essential oils used to improve mental concentration such as Peppermint, Eucalyptus, Lemon and Rosemary essential oils.

1 teaspoon dried ground herbs (optional) used to improve mental concentration such as rosemary leaves.

½ teaspoon colorant such as cocoa powder

Follow the above Basic Body Scrub Recipe Instructions.

***

Insomnia (Sleeplessness) Body Scrub Recipe

2 cups brown sugar

¾ cup or 6 oz or 190 ml of vegetable oils such as olive oil.

10 - 20 drops of essential oils such as Lavender, Roman chamomile, and Ylang ylang essential oils.

1 teaspoon dried ground herbs (optional) such as lavender flowers.

½ teaspoon colorant such as cocoa powder

Follow the above Basic Body Scrub Recipe Instructions.

***

Arthritis Body Scrub Recipe

2 cups brown sugar

¾ cup or 6 oz or 190 ml of vegetable oils with anti-inflammatory properties such as Pomegranate oil or Hemp seed oil. If you don't have these oils you can simply use olive oil.

10 - 20 drops of essential oils used for the treatment of arthritis such as Eucalyptus, Lemon, Lavender, Peppermint, Roman chamomile, and Rosemary essential oils.

1 teaspoon dried ground herbs (optional) used to manage arthritis such as arnica flowers, lavender flowers, rosemary leaves.

½ teaspoon colorant such as cocoa powder

Follow the above Basic Body Scrub Recipe Instructions.

***

Mosquito and Insect Repellant Body Scrub Recipe

2 cups brown sugar

¾ cup or 6 oz or 190 ml of vegetable oils such as olive oil.

10 - 20 drops of essential oils used to repel insects such as Eucalyptus, Lavender, Rosemary, and Geranium essential oils.

1 teaspoon dried ground herbs (optional) such as rosemary leaves and lavender flowers.

½ teaspoon colorant such as cocoa powder

Follow the above Basic Body Scrub Recipe Instructions.

* * * * *

5

Characteristics Of Vegetable Oils Used In Making Body Scrubs

Choose the vegetable oils you will use for your all natural body scrubs depending on your skin type and any other skin conditions you or your clients may be suffering from.

Sweet almond oil contains vitamins A, B, E, minerals and skin nourishing essential fatty acids. It is especially beneficial for normal skin, dry skin, sensitive skin, mature skin and eczema prone skin.

Sunflower oil contains vitamin A, E and skin nourishing essential fatty acids. It is especially beneficial for normal skin and dry skin.

Avocado oil is rich in skin nourishing nutrients. It is especially beneficial for normal skin, dry skin, sensitive skin, mature skin, eczema prone skin and psoriasis prone skin.

Apricot kernel oil contains vitamins A, E, minerals and skin nourishing essential fatty acids. It is especially beneficial for dry skin, sensitive skin, mature skin and prematurely aging skin. It is also useful for facial scrubs.

Jojoba is a plant wax which contains vitamin E, proteins, minerals and skin nourishing fatty acids and protective antioxidants. It is especially beneficial for normal skin, mature skin, oily or acne prone skin, eczema prone skin and psoriasis prone skin. It is also useful for facial scrubs.

Olive oil contains skin nourishing essential fatty acids and natural sunscreens. It is especially beneficial for dry skin, mature skin and eczema prone skin. It is also useful for hand scrubs since it conditions nails.

Evening primrose oil contains skin nourishing essential fatty acids, vitamins and minerals. It is especially beneficial for dry skin, mature skin, eczema prone skin and psoriasis prone skin.

Virgin coconut oil contains skin nourishing fatty acids. It is especially beneficial for dry skin. It is also useful for hand scrubs since it conditions nails.

Fractionated coconut oil is especially beneficial for dry skin and sensitive skin.

Canola oil is especially beneficial for normal skin, dry skin, sensitive skin and mature skin.

* * * * *

6

Characteristics Of Essential Oils Used In Making Body Scrubs

Choose the aromatherapy essential oils to use depending on the effects you want the body scrubs to have. For example:

Clary Sage Essential Oil has an herbaceous scent. It can help relieve stress related tension, reduce irritability and help one relax. It is also used for the management of mature and acne prone skin. Do not use it during pregnancy or if you are drinking alcohol or driving or if you have endometriosis, ovarian cysts, uterine cysts, breast cancer or you are at high risk for developing breast cancer as it may have an "estrogen-like" effect on the body.

Eucalyptus essential oil has an invigorating scent. It can help relieve stress related mental tension and mental exhaustion. It is also used in the management of joint aches and pains. Do not use eucalyptus essential oil if you have epilepsy, high blood pressure or apply it near a baby's nostrils.

Geranium Essential Oil has a fresh, minty rose scent. It can help relieve nervous tension and anxiety. It is also used in the management of eczema, cellulite as well as mature skin. Avoid using it in pregnancy.

Grapefruit essential oil has a refreshing, bitter-sweet scent. It can help relieve tension and release repressed emotions. It is also used in the management of cellulite.

Lavender essential oil has a soothing, floral scent. It can help one relax and relieve stress related tension, sleeplessness, anxiety and depression. It is also used in the management of acne, eczema and dry skin conditions. Do not use lavender essential oil in pregnancy, if you are breastfeeding, on young children as it may cause breast development in young boys and girls. Avoid it if you have low blood pressure as you may feel drowsy after using it.

Lemon essential oil has an clarifying fresh scent. It can help relieve mental tension, alleviate mental fatigue and increase concentration. It is also used in the management of acne and post acne dark skin spots. Do not use it if skin will be exposed to sunlight or UV rays in the next 12-24 hours. Do not use it if you have low blood pressure or you are allergic to lemons.

Lemongrass essential oil has a vitalizing, lemony scent. It can help relieve tension and muscle aches. It is also used in the management of acne. Do not use it if skin will be exposed to sunlight or UV rays in the next 12-24 hours.

Roman chamomile essential oil has a sweet and fruity scent. It can help relieve stress related tension headaches. It is also used in the management of eczema, psoriasis and dry skin conditions. Avoid using it in pregnancy and if you are allergic to ragweed.

Spearmint essential oil has a gently-energizing minty scent. It can help relieve mental tension and exhaustion. It is also used in the management of nausea.

Rosemary Essential Oil has an uplifting and stimulating scent. It can help relieve mental exhaustion and feeling rundown. It is also used in the management of eczema, muscle aches and joint pains. Do not use rosemary essential oil if you are pregnant or have epilepsy or high blood pressure. Avoid using it if you have a fever or you want to sleep and in children under 5 years.

Sweet orange essential oil has a cheeringly, refreshing scent. It can help mange stress related tension. It is also used in the management of cellulite and common colds. Do not use it if skin will be exposed to sunlight or UV rays in the next 12-24 hours.

Peppermint essential oil has a head-clearing, refreshing scent. It can help relieve tension and fatigue. It is also used to manage flatulence. Do not use peppermint essential oil in pregnancy, if breastfeeding, on children less than 5 years, if you have epilepsy or irregular heart beats or cardiac fibrillation or high blood pressure and before using a sun bed or going to hot humid places.

Tea tree essential oil has a purifying almost medicinal scent. It can help relieve tension and fatigue. It is also been used in the management of acne and athlete's foot.

Ylang ylang Essential Oil has a fragrantly floral scent. It can help relieve anxiety, tension and help one relax. It is also used as an aphrodisiac and in the management of dry skin conditions. Do not use ylang ylang essential oil if you have low blood pressure or sensitive, damaged skin.

* * * * *

7

Characteristics Of Herbs Used In Making Body Scrubs

Different herbs can be added to body scrubs to increase their esthetic appeal and healing benefits. These herbal healing benefits that will be extracted are as follows:

Arnica flowers are believed to have anti-inflammatory properties and are used to relieve the pains of sprains, muscle aches and joint pains. Do not use arnica if you are allergic to it, if pregnant or breastfeeding.

Calendula flowers are believed to have antioxidant, anti-inflammatory and anti-infective properties. They are used to help wounds heal faster, for minor cuts, small insect bites, minor bruises, first degree burns, mild sunburns and mild skin infections. Calendula has been shown to prevent dermatitis or skin inflammation in breast cancer patients receiving radiation treatment. Do not use calendula if you are allergic to it, allergic to daisy or aster family plants such as ragweed and chrysanthemums, if pregnant or breastfeeding or trying to conceive.

Avoid calendula preparations if you are taking sedatives, high blood pressure and diabetes medications.

Chamomile flowers are believed to have relaxing and mild antiseptic properties. They are used to help relieve anxiety, relieve emotional stress, relax tense muscles and relieve muscle spasms. Do not use/ avoid chamomile if you are allergic to it, allergic to daisy or aster family plants such as ragweed and chrysanthemums, have asthma, are pregnant as it may cause miscarriage, if driving as it may cause drowsiness, if taking alcohol, for at least 2 weeks before surgery or dental procedures as it may cause bleeding. Do not use/avoid chamomile if you are taking blood thinners such as warfarin (coumadin), clopidogrel (plavix) or aspirin as it may cause bleeding, sedatives, drugs used to treat sleeplessness, high blood pressure medications as it may lower the blood pressure and diabetes medications as it can lower the blood sugar.

Comfrey leaves are believed to have anti-inflammatory, skin regenerative and antiseptic properties. They are used to relieve muscle strains and ligament sprains. Do not use/ avoid comfrey if you are allergic to it, on broken skin, on children, the elderly, if pregnant or breastfeeding, in liver disease, alcoholism and cancer. Do not use/ avoid comfrey if you are taking acetaminophen (panadol, tylenol). Do not use/ avoid comfrey if using herbs known to cause liver problems such as kava, valerian and skullcap.

Lavender flowers are believed to have calming, analgesic, anti-inflammatory and skin regenerative properties. They are used to relieve tension, reduce anxiety, insomnia, manage eczema, muscle and joint aches. Do not use/ avoid lavender if you are allergic to it, on broken skin, if pregnant or breastfeeding, on young boys as it may cause male breast development. Do not use/ avoid lavender if you are taking sedatives, anti-anxiety medications such as lorazepam and narcotic analgesics such as morphine and oxycodone.

Rose petals are believed to have skin softening properties.

Rosemary leaves are believed to have antioxidant, mentally stimulating and antimicrobial properties. They are used to reduce feelings of sadness, increase mental concentration and relieve muscle pains and joint aches. Do not use/ avoid rosemary if you are allergic to it, are breastfeeding or pregnant as it may cause miscarriages, are under 18 years old, have high blood pressure, peptic ulcers, ulcerative colitis or Crohn's disease. Do not use/avoid rosemary if you are taking blood thinners such as warfarin (coumadin), clopidogrel (plavix) or aspirin as it may cause bleeding, angiotensin converting enzyme (ACE) inhibitors such as captopril and lisinopril for high blood pressure, diuretics such as furosemide (lasix) and hydrochlorothiazide also used for high blood pressure treatment and medicines for diabetes medications as it may alter the blood sugar levels and lithium.

St John's Wort flowers and leaves have anti-depressant, anti-inflammatory, antiseptic properties. They are used to relieve mild depression, and manage mild eczema. Do not use/ avoid St John's wort if you are allergic to it, have major or severe depression and bipolar disorder, are pregnant, breastfeeding or trying to get pregnant. Do not use/ avoid St John's wort if you are going to have surgery in five days, are taking digoxin for the heart, antiretroviral medicines used to treat HIV/ AIDS, if you are taking medications to treat depression as it could result in the dangerous serotonin syndrome. These antidepressant medications include serotonin reuptake inhibitors (SSRIs) such as citalopram, fluoxetine and sertraline, tricyclic antidepressants such as amitriptyline and imipramine, monoamine oxidase inhibitors (MAOIs) such as phenelzine and tranylcypromine.

* * * * *

8

Natural Colorants For Homemade Body Scrubs

You can use different natural substances to color your handmade homemade body scrubs.

For different shades of **brown** use honey, cinnamon, cocoa and coffee.

For different shades of **yellow** use calendula petals and yarrow.

For different shades of **red and pink** use paprika and cayenne pepper.

For different shades of **green** use French clay, powdered rosemary, sage and dried basil leaves.

For different shades of **orange** use turmeric.

* * * * *

About The Author

Dr. Miriam Kinai is a medical doctor and a certified aromatherapist.

You can visit her blog at
http://www.TheBestSellingEbooks.blogspot.com/

or follow her on twitter at http://twitter.com/AlmasiHealth

Email enquiries to drkinai@yahoo.com with BOOKS as your subject.

Other Books By Dr Miriam Kinai

Natural Body Products Series

Books in our Natural Body Product Series teach you how to make handmade bath and beauty products. They also teach you the benefits of various vegetable oils, essential oils, natural butters, and herbs to help you choose the best ingredients for your homemade products.

These books are filled with recipes for managing normal, sensitive, mature, and dry skin types as well as cellulite, eczema, psoriasis, ringworms, dandruff, thinning hair, menopause, pre-menstrual tension, painful periods, arthritis, stress, sadness, mental fatigue, and insomnia.

Books in the Natural Bath and Body Products Series include:

1. How to Make Handmade Natural Bath Bombs

2. How to Make Handmade Natural Bath Melts

3. How to Make Handmade Natural Bath Salts

4. How to Make Handmade Natural Bath Teas

5. How to Make Handmade Natural Body Butters

6. How to Make Handmade Natural Body Lotions

7. How to Make Handmade Natural Body Scrubs

8. How to Make Handmade Natural Healing Balms

9. How to Make Handmade Natural Herb Infused Oils

10. How to Make Handmade Natural Soap

* * * * *

Managing Stress with the Word of God

Managing Stress with the Word of God teaches you how to manage stress effectively by combining time tested Biblical principles with medical proven relaxation techniques.

Topics covered in this book include:

1. What is stress?

2. What is the body's response to stress?

3. Symptoms of Stress

4. Biblical Principles for Stress Management

5. Medical Relaxation Techniques

6. Other Stress Relief Activities

* * * * *

Rules Of Relaxation

Rules of Relaxation teaches you 130 simple relaxation techniques as it covers the A to Z of stress management from Assert yourself, Breathe deeply, Cast your burdens, Drink herbal teas, Establish social support, Formulate realistic goals, Guard your heart, Have complementary hobbies, Identify personal stressors, Jaunt, Keep the Sabbath, Listen to music, Meditate on the Word, Nab a nap, Optimize stress, Pamper yourself, Quash sin, Reason rationally, Schedule news fasts, Trust God, Use cognitive restructuring, Veto worry, Work out, eXperiment with aromatherapy, Yield to God to Zap job stress.

* * * * *

Sword Words

SWORD WORDS teaches you how to wage Christian spiritual warfare using the SWORD of the Spirit which is the WORD of God. (Ephesians 6:17)

It instructs you how to wield your SWORD WORDS together with the full armor of God. It demystifies the enemy's devices and explains the battle plan. It also tells you how to position yourself strategically and communicate effectively with your backup so that you can win your battles regardless of whether you are fighting for your marriage, children, or finances or fighting addictions, opposition, and fear.

* * * * *

Resolving Conflicts just like Jesus Christ

Resolving Conflicts just like Jesus Christ uses Biblical examples from Jesus Christ to King Solomon to teach Conflict Resolution Strategies, Third Party Mediation Techniques, Conflict Reduction and Prevention so that you can increase the peace in your home, the productivity of your ministry, and the profitability of your business.

* * * * *

Christian Anger Management

Christian Anger Management teaches Biblical anger management tips and self help strategies to help you manage anger instead of letting it manage you and destroy your testimony, life, family, and career.

* * * * *

Managing Stress For Teens

Managing Stress for Teens teaches teenagers Biblical principles, medical techniques, and life skills to manage 80 common teenage stressors.

It teaches them how to resist using alcohol, cigarettes, drugs, and how to overcome addiction. It edifies them to resist sexual temptation, fornication, pornography, homosexuality, and lesbianism. It also helps them cope with sickness, and disability.

Managing Stress for Teens also teaches teenagers how to manage emotions such as anger, anxiety, confusion, fear, guilt, loneliness, love, lust, low self confidence, and shyness. It guides them on how to deal with negative peer pressure. It also trains them to cope with family problems like abuse.

Managing Stress for Teens suggests constructive activities for teens who don't have money. It helps also helps them understand parental issues like pressure from parents and schools them on the best way to deal with bullying.

Managing Stress for Teens also clarifies issues on God, Jesus, The Holy Spirit, feeling they lack faith, and living right. It coaches them on how to deal with fashion trends, crime, corruption, and cultural practices. It also helps them understand puberty, their body shape, self image, gender realization and the effects of negative thoughts and words as well as helping them answer the questions "Who am I?" and "Why am I here?"

* * * * *

Dark Skin Dermatology Color Atlas

Dark Skin Dermatology Color Atlas is filled with clear explanations and color photos of skin, hair, and nail diseases affecting people with skin of color or Fitzpatrick skin types IV, V, and VI.

Topics covered include Acne Vulgaris, Alopecia Areata, Anal Warts, Angioedema, Aphthous Ulcers, Atopic Dermatitis, Blastomycosis, Blister Beetle Dermatitis or Nairobi Fly Dermatitis, Cellulitis, Chronic Ulcers, Confetti Hypopigmentation, Cutaneous T Cell Lymphoma, Cutaneous Tuberculosis, Dermatitis Artefacta, Erythema Nodosum, Exfoliative Erythroderma, Gianotti Crosti Syndrome, Hand Dermatitis , Hemangioma, Herpes Zoster, Ichthyosis, Ingrown Toenails, Irritant Contact Dermatitis, Kaposi Sarcoma, Keloids, Keratoderma Blenorrhagica, Klippel Trenaunay Weber Syndrome, Leishmaniasis, Leprosy, Leukonychia, Lichen Nitidus, Lichen Planus, Lichenoid Drug Eruption, Linear Epidermal Nevus, Linear IgA Dermatosis (LAD), Lipodermatosclerosis, Lymphangioma Circumscriptum, Miliaria, Molluscum Contagiosum, Neurofibromatosis, Nickel Dermatitis, Onychomadesis, Onychomycosis, Palmoplantar Eccrine Hidradenitis, Papular Pruritic Eruption (PPE), Paronychia, Pellagra, Pemphigus Foliaceous, Pemphigus Vulgaris, Piebaldism, Pityriasis Rosea, Pityriasis Rubra Pilaris, Plantar Hyperkeratosis, Plantar Warts, Poikiloderma, Postinflammatory Hyperpigmentation and Hypopigmentation, Post Topical Steroids Hypopigmentation, Psoriasis, Pyogenic Granuloma or Lobular Capillary Hemangioma, Scabies, Seborrheic Dermatitis, Steven Johnson Syndrome (SJS) and Toxic Epidermal Necrolysis (TEN), Sunburn, Systemic Sclerosis, Tinea Capitis, Tinea Pedis, Tinea Versicolor, Traction Alopecia, Urticaria, Vasculitis, Vitiligo, and Xanthelasma.

* * * * *

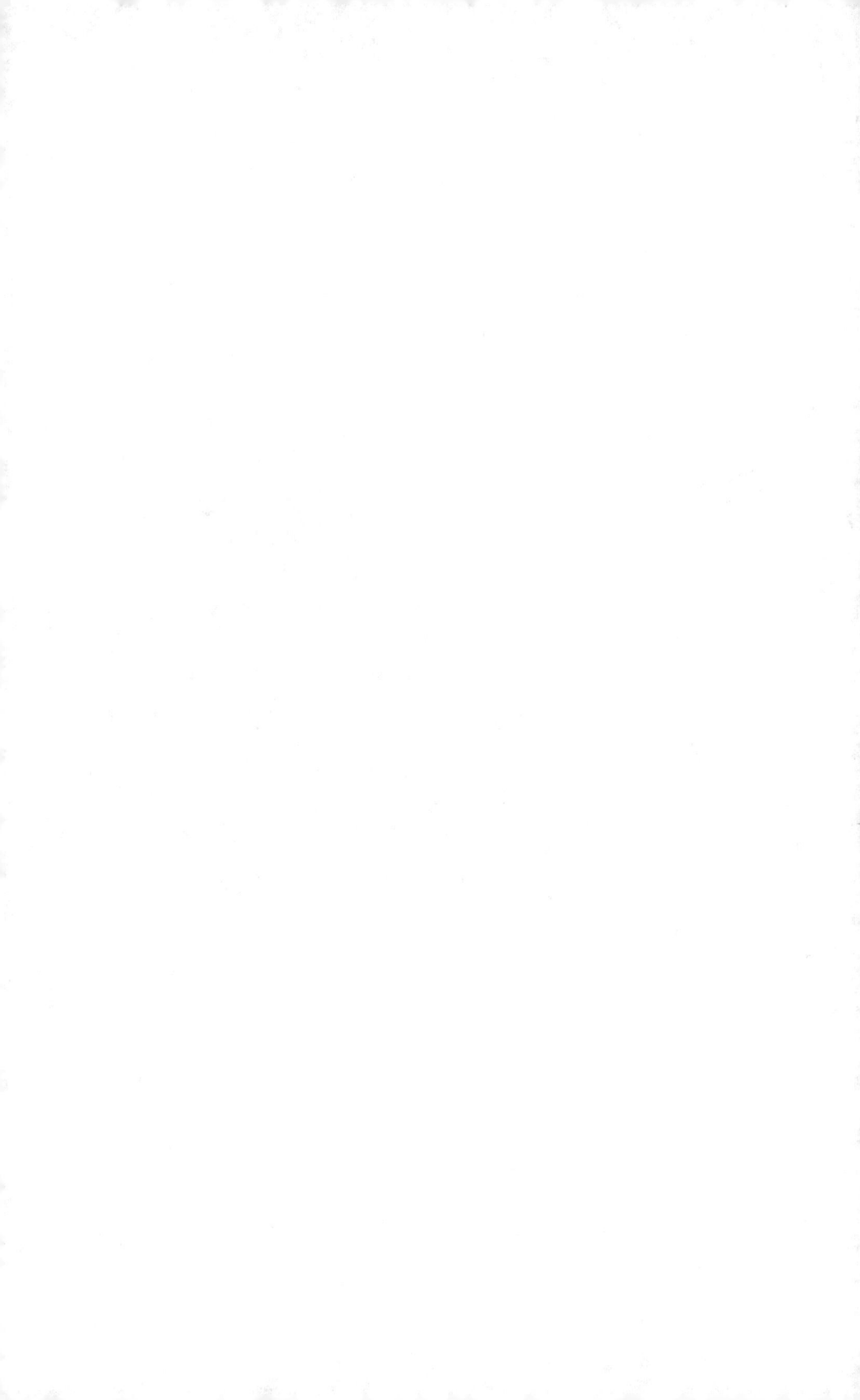